LOSE WEIGHT,

LOOK SEXY,

LIVE LONGER!

Inside This Book You'll Receive My
Exact Cardio, Nutrition, & Exercise
Regimen That I Use To Get
Guaranteed Results!

Stacy Mitchell

www.ChangeYourLifeOvernight.com

LOSE WEIGHT, LOOK SEXY, LIVE LONGER!
Inside This Book You'll Receive My Exact
Cardio, Nutrition, & Exercise Regimen That I
Use To Get Guaranteed Results!

TABLE OF CONTENTS:

I have included my greatest weight loss secrets of all time in this book. Not only that, but the information in this book can help cure you and your loved ones of any illness, sickness, and disease you currently might be experiencing. It's one thing to read a book, but it's another thing to do the things you learn in the book. If you want to lose weight, increase energy, cure illness, sickness, disease, and get into the best shape of your life, this is definitely the book for you. I put my name and reputation behind it.

Sincerely,
Stacy Mitchell

www.ChangeYourLifeOvernight.com

Chapter One:

Introduction.

Deciding to share my knowledge with the world and sell my most powerful weight loss secrets of all time is very gratifying, but also makes me a little bit jealous of you. You see, it took me a lot of trial, error, and studying to discover everything I'm about to share with you, but you're about to get everything by doing nothing more than paying a few dollars. It seems like you got the better deal. LOL.

Sometimes when we get something without putting in a lot of time, effort and money for it, we don't appreciate it as much. So, please do not take the weight loss secrets in this book for granted. Treasure them and put them to use every day just like I do. I can honestly say that I practice what I preach. My husband and I do every single thing that I'm going to share with you in the pages that follow. That's how we stay so fit, lean, sexy, energetic, and healthy.

This book could truly be worth a million dollars to you. Let me prove it to you by asking you a question. Why did you purchase this book?

To burn fat?

To live longer?

To lose weight?

To gain energy?

To sleep better?

To prevent heart disease?

To improve your memory?

To increase your strength?

To reduce your stress levels?

To eliminate your joint pain?

To heal yourself from cancer?

To lower your blood pressure?

To boost your immune system?

Now, let me ask you another question. If my secrets in this book help you achieve your goal how much would that be worth to you? $500? $1,000? $50,000? $100,000? What about one million dollars? If this book teaches you how to lose one hundred pounds of bodyfat, cure yourself of cancer, and gain more energy than you had when you were a teenager, how much money would that be worth to you? A lot of money right?

I have people from all over the world who write me testimonials telling me how much my weight loss secrets have changed their lives for the better. One man lost 150 pounds.

Another woman lost 70 pounds and cured herself of diabetes. Another man lost over 100 pounds and no longer has high blood pressure. Another woman was sad, depressed, overweight, recently divorced, and diagnosed with cancer, but now she's fit, happy, full of life, remarried, and completely healed of cancer.

These are only a few of the true life testimonials I've received from real people after they've put my weight loss secrets to work. This book will absolutely help you lose weight fast, and help you become much healthier in the process! Not only can the information in this book help you lose weight, but it could even save your life like it's already done for others.

So again, I hope you appreciate what you're about to discover and don't take this information for granted.

Based on the real life results that people all over the world are getting, I could have charged $10,000 for the information in this book, but I wanted to bless as many people as I possibly could and not have price be an issue.

I'm going to keep my weight loss secrets as short as I can to keep you from getting bored, but every piece of information I share with you is valuable. Put this information into daily use and tell me about the amazing results you achieve thirty days from now. God bless you!

Chapter Two:

Weight Loss Secrets.

Intermittent Fasting! To lose weight fast you want to start incorporating Intermittent Fasting into your daily lifestyle. In case you've never heard about Intermittent Fasting before let me give you some history about it so you can see the amazing benefits it can provide for you.

Intermittent Fasting is an eating pattern where you cycle between periods of eating and fasting. There are two different intermittent fasting methods, both of which split the day or week into eating periods and fasting periods.

Most people think of religion when they think of the word fasting. I know I first did. Throughout my child hood I had a friend in my neighborhood who would sometimes not eat when everyone else was. I would always ask him why he wasn't eating and he would always respond- I'm fasting.

Now granted, he was fasting as part of his religion, but today people are starting to fast more than ever before because of a lot of different health benefits. Here are just a few of the amazing health benefits you can receive from Intermittent Fasting:

-helps prevent cancer.

-reduces inflammation.

-benefits brain function.

-decreases insulin levels.

-boosts your metabolism.

-helps prevent Alzheimer's disease.

-removes waste material from cells.

-lowers your risk of getting diabetes.

-Insulin levels decrease significantly.

-lowers your risk of getting heart disease.

-Growth Hormone levels increase significantly.

-changes the function of cells, genes, and hormones.

-speeds up the fat burning and muscle building process.

-makes your stored body fat more accessible for energy.

-strengthens your immune system and helps you live a longer lifespan.

Did you read that? Intermittent Fasting will help you live LONGER!

If you've ever read The Holy Bible you can see that the people lived for 800 and 900 years. How is that possible and why is the average person only living about seventy-five years today?

Well, the people in The Holy Bible were actually doing Intermittent Fasting thousands of years ago. They would go days and weeks without eating. You'll notice that the people in The Holy Bible:

-Never Got Sick.

-Never Lacked Energy.

-Never Went To A Doctor.

-Never Ate Fast Food Or Sugar.

-Fasted For Days And Weeks At A Time.

-Walked (Exercised) Everywhere They Went.

-Had Lifespans That Lasted Hundreds And Hundreds Of Years.

So, Intermittent Fasting has been around since BC. However, our culture that we live in today has brainwashed us from the day we were born and most people are very close minded to trying something they haven't done before like Intermittent Fasting. The facts and results from thousands of years prove Intermittent Fasting works great for losing weight fast. I'm proof of that! Intermittent Fasting has not only changed my physical body on the outside, but it has truly changed my internal health as well. There's two main ways to do Intermittent Fasting:

-Choose two days per week and eat nothing on those two days. This is a twenty-four hour fast twice a week. This option requires two days per week without eating anything.

-Don't eat anything for sixteen hours of the day, every single day of the week. Eat all of your meals in an eight hour time period each day.

This second option is the option I live by. I eat all my meals every single day between 2pm-10pm. The remaining sixteen hours I don't eat anything.

Intermittent Fasting has a lot of health benefits, but the greatest two benefits it provides is the huge effect that it has on the production of two hormones in your body: Insulin and Growth Hormone.

Intermittent Fasting decreases your Insulin levels, which is good, because that means you're lowering your bodyfat percentage and able to lose weight faster.

Intermittent Fasting increases your Growth Hormone levels, which is good, because that means you're increasing your energy, your strength, and your muscle mass.

Lemon Water! Lemon Water will not only help you lose weight fast, but it has a lot of health healing benefits as well:

-reduces fever.

-kills cancer cells.

-cures indigestion.

-prevents diabetes.

-alkalizes the body.

-fights against acne.

-detoxifies the liver.

-dissolves gallstones.

-helps with regularity.

-prevents gum disease.

-neutralizes free radicals.

-increases oxygen supply.

-boosts the immune system.

-reduces high blood pressure.

-prevents Parkinson's disease.

-relieves respiratory problems.

On top of all of these health healing benefits, Lemon water also has some powerful weight loss properties as well. The weight loss effects of Lemon water are as follows:

-**increases your metabolism** by causing your body temperature to rise which allows the body to move fat into the bloodstream for the muscles to use for energy.

-**controls insulin levels** because it has a low glycemic index which is a measure of how much blood sugar levels rise after eating. By keeping your Insulin levels low you keep your body from storing food as fat.

-**lowers your cortisol levels** because it regulates the immune system and eases anxiety. Cortisol is a hormone that increases during times of stress and makes you fat, especially in the stomach area.

Do Cardio On An Empty Stomach! To lose weight fast you want to do your cardio first thing in the morning when you wake up on an empty stomach. Most people work a nine to five job and do cardio after they get off work at night. This is a problem because they've probably had three meals or so throughout the day, which means they have calories in their body when they get to the gym.

So, let's just say the average person does thirty minutes of cardio each day. Let's assume the average person burns five calories per minute. So, thirty minutes of cardio multiplied by five calories is a total of 150 calories that they burned during their cardio session. However, like I said before, they've probably had a few meals inside of them. So, the calories they burned didn't even touch their stored bodyfat. All they burned off was some of the calories they've already eaten. Yes, the cardio they did might help their heart stay in shape a little bit, but in regards to losing weight, which is what their goal of doing cardio is, this cardio session was a complete waste of time.

Now, let's start incorporating cardio first thing in the morning on an empty stomach and watch what happens. Let's just say the average person sleeps for eight hours per night. Let's assume the average person eats their last meal two hours before they go to sleep. So, when they wake up and do their cardio first thing in the morning on an empty stomach they haven't eaten anything for ten hours. This is exactly what you want to do. This is the perfect time to do your cardio and let me tell you the reason why.

Let's use the same scenario from before. The average person does thirty minutes of cardio each day. Let's assume the average person burns five calories per minute. So, thirty minutes of cardio multiplied by five calories is a total of 150 calories that they burned during their cardio session. However, this time the cardio was performed on an empty stomach. There were absolutely zero calories stored inside their body. So, the 150 calories that they burned didn't come from the meals they've already eaten, they came from stored bodyfat. This is how you lose weight.

If you've ever done your cardio after work like I described above, but didn't lose weight, now you know why. Start doing cardio first thing in the morning when you wake up on an empty stomach and your weight loss efforts will pay off immediately!

Cacao Powder (not Cocoa)! Cacao Powder will not only help you lose weight fast, but it has a lot of health healing benefits as well:

-improves libido.

-prevents sunburn.

-makes you happy.

-fights tooth decay.

-prevents blood clots.

-lowers blood pressure.

-causes better digestion.

-reduces type 2 diabetes.

-reduces the risk of stroke.

-reduces insulin resistance.

-stimulates bowel function.

-prevents premature aging.

-improves blood circulation.

-protects against skin cancer.

-strengthens your hair & nails.

-prevents Alzheimer's disease.

-protects against osteoporosis.

-restores feelings of well-being.

-protects against cardiovascular disease.

On top of all of these health healing benefits, Cacao Powder also has some powerful weight loss properties as well. The weight loss effects of Cacao Powder are as follows:

-**increases your energy** allowing you to burn more calories by working out harder and longer which will turn up thermogenesis in your body.

-**suppresses your appetite** by balancing your blood sugar levels and it improves the feeling of fullness because of the extremely high fiber content.

-**increases your metabolism** by causing your body temperature to rise, which allows the body to move fat into the bloodstream for the muscles to use for energy.

-**lowers your cortisol levels** because it regulates the immune system and eases anxiety. Cortisol is a hormone that increases during times of stress and makes you fat, especially in the stomach area.

Grapefruit! Grapefruit will not only help you lose weight fast, but it has a lot of health healing benefits as well:

-prevents asthma.

-prevents dehydration.

-prevents constipation.

-helps fight skin damage.

-decreases the risk of stroke.

-decreases the risk of cancer.

-reduces high blood pressure.

-decreases the risk of diabetes.

-decreases the risk of heart disease.

-protects against loss of muscle mass.

-reduces the formation of kidney stones.

On top of all of these health healing benefits, Grapefruit also has some powerful weight loss properties as well. The weight loss effects of Grapefruit are as follows:

-**reduces insulin levels** which means your body can more efficiently use food for energy rather than storing it as fat.

-**suppresses your appetite** by increasing blood flow which increases the amount of calories you burn while making you feel full so you eat less.

-**increases your metabolism** by causing your body temperature to rise which allows the body to move fat into the bloodstream for the muscles to use for energy.

Coconut Oil! Coconut Oil will not only help you lose weight fast, but it has a lot of health healing benefits as well:

-kills cancer.

-heals arthritis.

-improves digestion.

-reduces pancreatitis.

-treats yeast infections.

-prevents gum disease.

-reduces inflammation.

-prevents osteoporosis.

-prevents heart disease.

-boosts immune system.

-prevents premature aging.

-improves type 2 Diabetes.

-heals many skin disorders.

-treats Alzheimer's disease.

-clears up kidney infections.

-reduces high blood pressure.

-heals urinary tract infections.

-naturally balances hormones.

-improves memory & brain function.

On top of all of these health healing benefits, Coconut Oil also has some powerful weight loss properties as well. The weight loss effects of Coconut Oil are as follows:

-**increases your energy** allowing you to burn more calories by working out harder and longer which will turn up thermogenesis in your body.

-**suppresses your appetite** by increasing blood flow which increases the amount of calories you burn while making you feel full so you eat less.

-**increases your metabolism** from all of the Medium Chain Triglycerides. MCT's are metabolized differently than the longer chain fats and MCT's are sent straight to the liver from the digestive tract where they're used for energy right away.

Honey! Honey will not only help you lose weight fast, but it has a lot of health healing benefits as well:

-heals acne.

-disinfects cuts.

-improves sleep.

-relieves herpes.

-boosts memory.

-increases energy.

-body moisturizer.

-helps with eczema.

-fights gum disease.

-increases sex drive.

-suppresses coughs.

-soothes acid reflux.

-helps prevent cancer.

-treats yeast infections.

-helps with cholesterol.

-reduces allergy symptoms.

-strengthens your immune system.

On top of all of these health healing benefits, Honey also has some powerful weight loss properties as well. The weight loss effects of Honey are as follows:

-**releases fat burning hormones** because the liver produces glucose which keeps the brain sugar levels high.

-**lowers your cortisol levels** by having a calming effect on the body it activates the recovery hormone melatonin that is exclusively for fat burning.

-**increases your metabolism** by causing your body temperature to rise, which burns fat for energy.

Drink Caffeine During Your Workouts! To lose weight fast you want to drink caffeine during your workouts. I've been doing this with my husband for years and it's played a big role in my body staying lean and sexy every single day of the year.

I personally drink one can of sugar free, calorie free Monster during my workouts. Make sure whatever your caffeine beverage of choice is that it doesn't contain any sugar or calories. Drinking sugar and calories would totally defeat the purpose of trying to lose weight. Drinking caffeine during your workouts helps you lose weight in two different ways:

-**increases your metabolism** because it jumpstarts the process of lipolysis which is when your body releases free fatty acids into the bloodstream. This occurs when your body is breaking down your fat stores to convert them into energy.

-**increases your energy** because caffeine is a stimulant. It allows you to burn more calories by working out harder and longer, which will turn up thermogenesis in your body. It also increases alertness and wards off drowsiness, which means that you can perform certain tasks for longer. This includes physical tasks such as cardio and lifting weights. This means a little shot of caffeine can give you the energy you need to give 100% effort during your workouts.

Ground Cinnamon! Ground Cinnamon will not only help you lose weight fast, but it has a lot of health healing benefits as well:

-freshens breath.

-reduces risk of cancer.

-reduces inflammation.

-relieves muscle soreness.

-lowers blood sugar levels.

-fights against tooth decay.

-prevents premature aging.

-cures candida overgrowth.

-boosts your immune system.

-reduces free radical damage.

-reduces risk of heart disease.

-protects skin from irritations.

-reduces symptoms of allergies.

-fights against harmful infections.

-reduces risk of Parkinson's disease.

-reduces risk of Alzheimer's disease.

On top of all of these health healing benefits, Ground Cinnamon also has some powerful weight loss properties as well. The weight loss effects of Ground Cinnamon are as follows:

-**suppresses your appetite** by increasing blood flow which increases the amount of calories you burn while making you feel full so you eat less.

-**lowers your cortisol levels** by having a calming effect on the body it activates the recovery hormone melatonin that is exclusively for fat burning.

-**increases your metabolism** because it jumpstarts the process of lipolysis, which is when your body releases free fatty acids into the bloodstream. This occurs when your body is breaking down your fat stores to convert them into energy.

-**controls insulin levels** by imitating the activity of insulin in the body. Insulin is the chemical that helps your body regulate its levels of blood sugar. Increased blood sugar levels can be problematic because they cause excess fat to be stored in the body making it harder for people to lose weight. Cinnamon helps regulate your blood sugar levels so this excess fat does not build up.

Ground Flaxseed! Ground Flaxseed will not only help you lose weight fast, but it has a lot of health healing benefits as well:

-heals acne.

-lowers cholesterol.

-improves blood sugar.

-reduces inflammation.

-reduces sugar cravings.

-cuts hot flashes in half.

-promotes digestive health.

-eliminates yeast and candida.

-supports colon detoxification.

-reduces the risk of osteoporosis.

-reduces the risk of all kinds of cancer.

-reduces dryness in your skin and hair.

-reduces the risk of cardiovascular disease.

On top of all of these health healing benefits, Ground Flaxseed also has some powerful weight loss properties as well. The weight loss effects of Ground Flaxseed are as follows:

-**suppresses your appetite** by increasing blood flow which increases the amount of calories you burn while making you feel full so you eat less.

-**protects against metabolic syndrome** by lowering blood levels of lipids and glucose. Their potential to reduce glucose will help you lose weight.

-**controls insulin levels** because they have a low glycemic index which is a measure of how much blood sugar levels rise after eating.

Ground Turmeric (Curcumin)!
Ground Turmeric will not only help you lose weight fast, but it has a lot of health healing benefits as well:

-prevents cancer.

-improves memory.

-lowers blood sugar.

-reduces inflammation.

-treats high cholesterol.

-decreases arthritis pain.

-fights against depression.

-reverses type 2 Diabetes.

-prevents premature aging.

-lowers risk of heart disease.

-prevents Alzheimer's disease.

-neutralizes damaging free radicals.

On top of all of these health healing benefits, Ground Turmeric also has some powerful weight loss properties as well. The weight loss effects of Ground Turmeric are as follows:

-**boosts your metabolism** by fastening to capsaicin receptors and increases thermogenesis which leads to greater fat burning.

-**lowers cortisol levels** by having a calming effect on the body it activates the recovery hormone melatonin that is exclusively fat burning.

-**controls insulin levels** which is a measure of how much blood sugar levels rise after eating. By keeping your Insulin levels low you keep your body from storing food as fat.

-**helps you block fat** by inhibiting the formation of fatty tissue.

Wear Sweats During Your Workouts!
To lose weight fast you want to cover your entire body by wearing sweats during your workouts. I've been doing this for years and it's played a big role in my body staying lean and sexy every single day of the year.

Wearing sweats from head to toe during your workouts helps you lose weight by trapping your body heat underneath the clothing. The body heat can't escape the clothing. This increases thermogenesis in the body helping you to burn more calories in a shorter period of time.

As of this writing I'm currently living in Columbus, Ohio. It's winter time and yesterday I went outside to go running even though it was zero degrees. I had three layers of sweats on. Even though it was zero degrees outside, underneath my clothing I was actually sweating. This proves you will burn more calories covering your body in sweats during your workouts, even if you're working out in zero degree weather.

Ground Cayenne Pepper! Ground Cayenne Pepper will not only help you lose weight fast, but it has a lot of health healing benefits as well:

-relieves gas.

-heals the flu.

-relieves joint pain.

-detoxifies the body.

-heals upset stomach.

-prevents lung cancer.

-helps relieve allergies.

-reduces atherosclerosis.

-stimulates the digestive tract.

-prevents migraine headaches.

-stimulates the circulatory system.

-breaks up mucus and inflammation.

-keeps blood pressure levels normal.

-fights tooth decay and gum disease.

On top of all of these health healing benefits, Ground Cayenne Pepper also has some powerful weight loss properties as well. The weight loss effects of Ground Cayenne Pepper are as follows:

-**increases fat oxidation** by increasing your body's heat production.

-**suppresses your appetite** by increasing blood flow which increases the amount of calories you burn while making you feel full so you eat less.

-**increases your metabolism** by causing your body temperature to rise which allows the body to move fat into the bloodstream for the muscles to use for energy.

Apple Cider Vinegar! Apple Cider Vinegar will not only help you lose weight fast, but it has a lot of health healing benefits as well:

-whitens teeth.

-heals sunburn.

-removes warts.

-kills cancer cells.

-clears out sinuses.

-heals sore throats.

-lowers cholesterol.

-detoxifies the liver.

-lowers blood sugar.

-heals upset stomach.

-promotes circulation.

-eliminates bad breath.

-healthy salad dressing.

-can be used as deodorant.

-gives you soft and shiny hair.

-prevents acne as a face wash.

On top of all of these health healing benefits, Apple Cider Vinegar also has some powerful weight loss properties as well. The weight loss effects of Apple Cider Vinegar are as follows:

-**reduces water retention** by replenishing potassium in the body to help reduce sodium levels.

-**suppresses your appetite** by balancing your blood sugar levels and improves the feeling of fullness.

-**increases your metabolism** by having an alkaline effect on your body and speeds up weight loss.

HIIT (High Intensity Interval Training)! To lose weight fast you want to do HIIT for your cardio. HIIT is a way of doing cardio with short bursts of high intensity energy (exercising) followed by short bursts of low intensity energy (resting).

HIIT is designed to get your heart rate elevated very quickly for a minute or two, then bringing your heart rate back down to normal by resting for a minute or two. If you did a cardio session for twenty minutes with one minute intervals then your actual cardio (exercise) time would only be ten minutes long.

Can you imagine doing only ten minutes of cardio a few days a week and losing weight effortlessly? Believe me, it's possible! Let me give you an example of a HIIT session:

Let's say you're using the treadmill for a twenty-minute cardio session. Let's say you run really quickly (exercise) for one minute, followed by walking slowly (resting) for one minute. You would do this interval sequence of one minute fast followed by one minute slow the entire twenty minutes.

Cardio goes by very quickly when you do HIIT. Not only that, but what makes HIIT so powerful for losing weight is the after burn effect. The after burn effect is all the calories you burn after your cardio session is over.

You see, by getting your heart rate up for one minute, then bringing it back down for one minute, followed by taking it back up for one minute, then bringing it back down for one minute, you're actually confusing your heart rate. It doesn't know whether to go up or go down. So, after your twenty-minute cardio session is over, the weight loss process is far from being over. The weight loss process has only just begun because since you confused your heart rate your body is going to continue to burn fat for the next twenty-four hours straight, even while you're sleeping!

You'll start noticing every morning when you get out of bed that you're leaner than you were the night before. This is because your body was burning calories all night long while you were sleeping. That's the amazing benefit of doing HIIT type cardio sessions. With HIIT you get to burn a lot more calories by doing a lot less cardio.

Chia Seeds! Chia Seeds will not only help you lose weight fast, but they have a lot of health healing benefits as well:

-kills cancer cells.

-fights bad breath.

-strengthens bones.

-regulates cholesterol.

-lowers blood pressure.

-reduces inflammation.

-balances insulin levels.

-reduces type 2 diabetes.

-prevents premature aging.

-promotes bowel regularity.

On top of all of these health healing benefits, Chia Seeds also have some powerful weight loss properties as well. The weight loss effects of Chia Seeds are as follows:

-**increases your metabolism** by having an alkaline effect on your body and speeds up weight loss.

-**suppresses your appetite** by balancing your blood sugar levels and improves the feeling of fullness.

-**lowers cortisol levels** by having a calming effect on the body it activates the recovery hormone melatonin that is exclusively fat burning.

Eat Apples! Eating apples will not only help you lose weight fast, but they have a lot of health healing benefits as well:

-cures constipation.

-detoxifies your liver.

-reduces tooth decay.

-strengthens your heart.

-lowers cholesterol levels.

-reduces the risk of stroke.

-reduces the risk of cancer.

-reduces the risk of diabetes.

-boosts your immune system.

-fights against Alzheimer's disease.

-protects against Parkinson's disease.

On top of all of these health healing benefits, Apples also have some powerful weight loss properties as well. The weight loss effects of Apples are as follows:

-**increases your energy** allowing you to burn more calories by working out harder and longer which will turn up thermogenesis in your body.

-**suppresses your appetite** by increasing blood flow which increases the amount of calories you burn while making you feel full so you eat less.

-**controls insulin levels** because they have a low glycemic index which is a measure of how much blood sugar levels rise after eating. By keeping your Insulin levels low you keep your body from storing food as fat.

Green Juice! Green Juice will not only help you lose weight fast, but it has a lot of health healing benefits as well:

-reduces pain.

-reduces nausea.

-fights infections.

-lowers blood sugar.

-improves digestion.

-cures stomach ulcers.

-helps prevent cancer.

-reduces osteoarthritis.

-reduces inflammation.

-improves heart disease.

-reduces menstrual pain.

-improves brain function.

-reduces type 2 diabetes.

-lowers cholesterol levels.

-reduces muscle soreness.

-treats chronic indigestion.

-boosts the immune system.

-protects against Heart disease.

-cleanses the lymphatic system.

-protects against Alzheimer's disease.

On top of all of these health healing benefits, Green Juice also has some powerful weight loss properties as well. The weight loss effects of Green Juice are as follows:

-**suppresses your appetite** by increasing blood flow which increases the amount of calories you burn while making you feel full so you eat less.

-**increases your metabolism** by causing your body temperature to rise which allows the body to move fat into the bloodstream for the muscles to use for energy.

-lowers your cortisol levels because it regulates the immune system and eases anxiety. Cortisol is a hormone that increases during times of stress and makes you fat, especially in the stomach area.

You can get Green Juice here: www.LoseWeightProtein.com

Black Beans! Black Beans will not only help you lose weight fast, but they have a lot of health healing benefits as well:

-shrinks tumors.

-increases energy.

-alkalizes the body.

-improves digestion.

-fights against cancer.

-builds healthy bones.

-reduces inflammation.

-lowers high cholesterol.

-reduces type 2 diabetes.

-prevents premature aging.

-promotes bowel regularity.

-reduces high blood pressure.

-prevents erectile dysfunction.

-protects against Heart disease.

-strengthens the immune system.

-protects against Parkinson's disease.

-protects against Alzheimer's disease.

-protects against Cardiovascular disease.

On top of all of these health healing benefits, Black Beans also have some powerful weight loss properties as well. The weight loss effects of Black Beans are as follows:

-**increases your energy** allowing you to burn more calories by working out harder and longer which will turn up thermogenesis in your body.

-**suppresses your appetite** by balancing your blood sugar levels and improves the feeling of fullness because of the high fiber content.

-**controls insulin levels** because they have a low glycemic index which is a measure of how much blood sugar levels rise after eating. By keeping your Insulin levels low you keep your body from storing food as fat.

Eat Oatmeal! Eating Oatmeal will not only help you lose weight fast, but it has a lot of health healing benefits as well:

-increases energy.

-helps relieve eczema.

-helps prevent asthma.

-lowers high cholesterol.

-reduces type 2 diabetes.

-reduces the risk of cancer.

-helps relieve constipation.

-promotes bowel regularity.

-reduces high blood pressure.

-reduces the risk of heart attack.

-strengthens the immune system.

-protects against Cardiovascular disease.

On top of all of these health healing benefits, Oatmeal also has some powerful weight loss properties as well. The weight loss effects of Oatmeal are as follows:

-**increases your energy** allowing you to burn more calories by working out harder and longer which will turn up thermogenesis in your body.

-**suppresses your appetite** by balancing your blood sugar levels and improves the feeling of fullness because of the high fiber content.

-**controls insulin levels** because they have a low glycemic index which is a measure of how much blood sugar levels rise after eating. By keeping your Insulin levels low you keep your body from storing food as fat.

Ground Nutmeg! Ground Nutmeg will not only help you lose weight fast, but it has a lot of health healing benefits as well:

-relieves arthritis.

-reduces insomnia.

-relieves joint pain.

-kills leukemia cells.

-detoxifies the body.

-soothes indigestion.

-reduces constipation.

-helps treat dementia.

-eliminates bad breath.

-lowers blood pressure.

-boosts immune system.

-dissolves kidney stones.

-improves blood circulation.

-strengthens cognitive function.

On top of all of these health healing benefits, Ground Nutmeg also has some powerful weight loss properties as well. The weight loss effects of Ground Nutmeg are as follows:

-**breaks down fats & cholesterol** which is an important process in losing weight because of its high levels of manganese.

-**suppresses your appetite** by balancing your blood sugar levels and improves the feeling of fullness because of the high fiber content.

Horseradish! Horseradish will not only help you lose weight fast, but it has a lot of health healing benefits as well:

-prevents cancer.

-increases energy.

-reduces joint pain.

-fights off infection.

-detoxifies the liver.

-improves digestion.

-heals sinus infections.

-prevents constipation.

-reduces inflammation.

-lowers blood pressure.

-prevents heart disease.

-boosts immune system.

-improves concentration.

-reduces water retention.

-relieves urinary infections.

-eliminates nasal congestion.

-reduces risk of osteoporosis.

-increases nutritional absorption.

-eliminates risk of neural tube defects.

On top of all these health healing benefits, Horseradish also has some powerful weight loss properties as well. The weight loss effects of Horseradish are as follows:

-**suppresses your appetite** by balancing your blood sugar levels and improves the feeling of fullness.

-**increases your energy** allowing you to burn more calories by working out harder and longer which will turn up thermogenesis in your body.

-**acts as a diuretic** by reducing water retention. The root is a natural diuretic, which helps to improve urine flow flushing fluids out of the body.

Resistance Training With Weights!
To lose weight fast you want to start incorporating resistance training into your lifestyle. In case you've never trained with weights before let me give you a little history.

Resistance training is the use of resistance to muscular contraction to help a person burn fat, lose weight, increase strength, boost energy, and build lean muscle mass. There are four different forms of resistance training: free weights, resistance bands, weighted machines, and your own bodyweight.

Resistance training will not only help you lose weight fast, but it has a lot of health healing benefits as well:

-reduces insomnia.

-improves posture.

-strengthens joints.

-improves flexibility.

-boosts energy levels.

-improves your mood.

-protects bone health.

-increases confidence.

-increases sperm count.

-decreases arthritis pain.

-alleviates low back pain.

-sharpens concentration.

-reduces type 2 diabetes.

-fights against depression.

-improves blood circulation.

-lowers high blood pressure.

-prevents erectile dysfunction.

-decreases risk of osteoporosis.

-strengthens the immune system.

-improves balance & coordination.

On top of all of these health healing benefits resistance training also has some powerful weight loss properties as well. The weight loss effects of resistance training are as follows:

-**increases fat oxidation** by increasing your body's heat production.

-**increases your metabolism** by replacing bodyfat with lean muscle because muscle burns more calories than fat.

-**releases fat burning hormones** because of the increase in your natural testosterone & growth hormone levels.

-**increases your energy** which will turn up thermogenesis in your body.

Chapter Three:

My Daily Dietary Regimen.

I hope you've enjoyed receiving this information as much as I've enjoyed giving it to you! Now you need to start incorporating it into your daily lifestyle. To keep you from getting confused or overwhelmed I'm going to include my personal daily dietary regimen for you below. If you want to follow my regimen for yourself you're more than welcome to. Or, if you just want to use it as a guideline that is perfectly fine as well.

Let me show you exactly how I incorporate every single one of my weight loss secrets into my daily lifestyle and how you can too. Once you get into the habit of working these into your lifestyle you won't ever have to think about it again.

As soon as I wake up in the morning:

I swallow 1 tbs of Coconut Oil.

I swallow 2 capsules of Korean Ginseng.

I gulp down ¼ cup of Apple Cider Vinegar.

I then drink my fat melting Hot Chocolate, which contains:

2 tbs of Cacao Powder.

4 tbs of Raw Honey.

1 tsp of Ground Cinnamon.

1 tsp of Ground Turmeric.

1 tsp of Ground Nutmeg.

Thirty minutes after I wake up in the morning, I go to the gym and do my cardio and resistance training on an empty stomach. I cover myself in sweats and I drink one can of sugar free Monster during my workout.

I eat an Intermittent Fasting lifestyle for all my meals. I consume all my food between 2pm-10pm.

Meal 1 at 2:00 pm:

2 tbs of Flaxseed.

2 tbs of Chia Seeds.

2 servings of Fresh Fruit.

1 cup of Gluten Free Oatmeal.

Mix all ingredients in a bowl with hot water.

Meal 2 at 5:00 pm: protein smoothie.

Mix the following in a Vitamix:

Spinach, Cucumber, Apple, Pineapple, Strawberries, Blueberries, & Honey.

2 scoops of Complete Protein.

24oz of cold water.

You can get Complete Protein here: www.LoseWeightProtein.com

Meal 3 at 8:00 pm: salad.

Mix the following in a bowl:

Spinach, Tomato, Black Beans, Veggie Burger, Tortilla Chips, Apple Cider Vinegar for a dressing.

Before I go to sleep at night:

I drink my fat melting Hot Chocolate, which contains:

2 tbs of Cacao Powder.

4 tbs of Raw Honey.

1 tsp of Ground Cinnamon.

1 tsp of Ground Turmeric.

1 tsp of Ground Nutmeg.

I also drink one gallon of water filled with Lemons every day. This gives me energy, helps me lose bodyfat, and strengthens my immune system.

I have perfect health! I haven't been to a Doctor in over twenty years. I don't smoke, drink, or do any drugs whatsoever. This includes both pharmaceutical and recreational. I've had a single digit bodyfat percentage for over twenty years now. So, like I said in the beginning, do not take these weight loss secrets for granted. They work big time!

What I just shared with you will not only help you lose weight faster than anything else in the world, but it will also help you live a longer and healthier lifespan.

I hope you not only enjoyed this information, but learned some very valuable secrets that can truly change your life forever. I love hearing about the success people have. Consider me your friend and your coach. Please stay in touch with me. Share your personal testimony with me once you achieve it. If you have any questions, or if there's anything else I can do to help you reach your health and fitness goals, please contact me anytime. I wish you nothing but the best of success! God bless you!

Chapter Four:

Exercise Routines.

Whether you're a professional athlete, or someone who is 100 pounds overweight and never worked out a day in your life, my weight loss secrets will help you lose weight faster than anything else on the market today. Since people of many different levels of physical fitness will buy this book, I'm going to lay out three different exercise regimens so you can follow the one that's best suited for you.

If you consider yourself to be at the **Beginner** level (you have a lot of weight to lose and you don't know much about working out) then I encourage you to follow this walking exercise routine I've put together for you. This will allow you to get some exercise, but nothing too strenuous that you can't follow through with.

Beginner level exercise routine:

Monday: 20 minutes of interval based walking. I want you to walk very quickly for 1 minute, then I want you to walk very slowly for 1 minute. I want you to do this for 20 minutes. Congratulate yourself when you're done! You are now one day closer to reaching your ultimate weight loss goal.

Wednesday: 20 minutes of interval based walking. I want you to walk very quickly for 1 minute, then I want you to walk very slowly for 1 minute. I want you to do this for 20 minutes. Congratulate yourself when you're done! You are now one day closer to reaching your ultimate weight loss goal.

Friday: 20 minutes of interval based walking. I want you to walk very quickly for 1 minute, then I want you to walk very slowly for 1 minute. I want you to do this for 20 minutes. Congratulate yourself when you're done! You are now one day closer to reaching your ultimate weight loss goal.

You can substitute another form of cardio for walking if you want to. Switch it up sometimes and do the treadmill one day, the stationary bike one day and the elliptical one day. That's 3 different workouts per week. Every single 20 minute cardio session you complete you're getting yourself closer to your ultimate weight loss goal.

Just take it one day at a time. As you begin to lose weight and gain mobility you can then move up to the

Intermediate level routine. Congratulations! I'm proud of you!

If you consider yourself to be at the **Intermediate** level (you've worked out before, you might even belong to a gym, but you're not very comfortable lifting weights by yourself) then I encourage you to follow this machine based exercise routine I've put together for you.

Intermediate level exercise routine: ALL exercises are on machines.

Monday: Chest, Shoulders & Triceps.

Seated Chest Press: 3 sets by 20, 15, 12 (add weight each set).

Seated Shoulder Press: 3 sets by 20, 15, 12 (add weight each set).

Seated Tricep Press: 3 sets by 20, 15, 12 (add weight each set).

Wednesday: Quadriceps, Hamstrings, Glutes & Calves.

Seated Leg Press: 3 sets by 20, 15, 12 (add weight each set).

Seated Leg Curl: 3 sets by 20, 15, 12 (add weight each set).

Seated Leg Extension: 3 sets by 20, 15, 12 (add weight each set).

Leg Press Calf Raises: 3 sets by 20, 15, 12 (add weight each set).

Friday: Back, Biceps & Forearms.

Lat Pulldown: 3 sets by 20, 15, 12 (add weight each set).

Seated Row: 3 sets by 20, 15, 12 (add weight each set).

Seated Curls: 3 sets by 20, 15, 12 (add weight each set).

Each day that you workout you're getting closer to reaching your goals. Just take it one day at a time. You're on your way to losing weight, sculpting lean muscle, and making your way to the advanced free weights. Congratulations! I'm proud of you!

If you consider yourself to be at the **Advanced** level (this means you exercise regularly, you're comfortable working out with free weights by yourself, and you only have 10-20 pounds to lose) then I encourage you to follow this free weight exercise routine I've put together for you.

Advanced level exercise routine:

Deadlifts- The Entire Body

Dips- Chest, Shoulders & Triceps

Pull Ups- Back, Biceps & Forearms

Barefoot Barbell Calf Raises- Calves

Lying Leg Curls- Hamstrings & Calves

Push Ups- Chest, Shoulders & Triceps

Leg Presses- Quadriceps, Hamstrings & Glutes

Bicep Curls (DB or Barbell)- Biceps & Forearms

Shoulder Presses (DB or Barbell)- Shoulders & Triceps

Deep Barbell Squats- Quadriceps, Hamstrings & Glutes

Bench Presses (DB or Barbell)- Chest, Shoulders & Triceps

The above exercises are the cream of the crop for losing weight and sculpting lean muscle mass!

Monday: Chest, Shoulders & Triceps.

Push Ups: 3 sets to failure (bodyweight only).

Barbell Bench Presses: 4 sets by 20, 15, 12, 8 (add weight each set).

Seated Barbell Presses: 3 sets by 15, 12, 8 (add weight each set).

Wednesday: Quadriceps, Hamstrings, Glutes & Calves.

Leg Presses: 4 sets by 20, 15, 12, 8 (add weight each set).

Lying Leg Curls: 3 sets by 20, 15, 12 (add weight each set).

Barefoot Barbell Calf Raises: 2 sets by 20, 15 (add weight each set).

Friday: Back, Biceps & Forearms.

Deadlifts: 3 sets by 15, 12, 8 (add weight each set).

Lat Pulldown: 3 sets by 20, 15, 12 (add weight each set).

Seated DB Curls: 3 sets by 15, 12, 8 (add weight each set).

Every workout that you complete brings you another pound closer to reaching your goals. There will be days when you don't feel like working out, but stay committed to reaching your goals and the results you achieve will be well worth it. Congratulations! I'm proud of you!

Chapter Five:

Sexy Sculpted Stomach.

Everyone wants a lean, sexy, sculpted stomach. It's what we all strive for. Not only does our health improve drastically by not having to carry around all that extra belly fat, but it feels good to look in the mirror and see ripples in your stomach. So, I'm going to teach you the only three abdominal exercises you'll ever need to know to get that dream stomach.

The good thing is just like cardio you do not have to do a lot of abdominal exercises to get a lean, sexy, sculpted stomach. You see, you have a six pack right now. It just might be covered under a layer of fat. Doing crunches all day long isn't going to burn that bodyfat off at all.

My weight loss secrets are going to burn all the bodyfat off and give you a lean, sexy, sculpted stomach.

The resistance training, or the abdominal exercises are just going to build a strong abdominal wall so that when your bodyfat is low enough your abs will be lean, sexy and sculpted. There are only three abdominal exercises that I ever do and they're the same three exercises I encourage you to do. These three exercises focus on all four areas of the abdominal wall:

Transversus Abdominis: the deepest muscle layer. Its main roles are to stabilize the trunk and maintain internal abdominal pressure.

Rectus Abdominis: this is slung between the ribs and the pubic bone at the front of the pelvis. When contracting this muscle it has the characteristic bumps or bulges that are commonly called "six pack". The main function of the rectus abdominis is to move the body between the ribcage and the pelvis.

External Oblique Muscles: these are on both sides of the rectus abdominis. The external oblique muscles allow the trunk to twist, but to the opposite side of whichever external oblique is contracting. For example, the right external oblique contracts to turn the body to the left.

Internal Oblique Muscles: these flank the rectus abdominis and are located just inside the hipbones. They operate in the opposite way to the external oblique muscles. For example, twisting the trunk to the left requires the left side internal oblique and the right side external oblique to contract together.

The three exercises that work all four areas of the abdominal wall are:

1. **Lying Leg Raises**: lay down on a decline bench. Your head is at the higher side of the bench with your feet at the lower side of the bench. Reach up behind with your hands and grab hold of the bench keeping your arms in close to your head. With your toes pointed up toward you, your feet slightly apart from each other, and your knees straight, raise your feet straight up about 12 inches (this is the midpoint). Hold for one second while squeezing your abs hard. Then slowly lower your feet to the starting position. Repeat this until failure.

2. **Hanging Leg Raises**: hold onto a bar above your head. Let your legs hang straight down. Without rocking or swaying your hips raise your feet up so that they're parallel to the

floor. While your legs are parallel (this is the midpoint) squeeze your abs hard for one second. Then slowly lower your feet to the starting position. Repeat this until failure.

3. **Parallel Bar Dip Leg Raises**: hold onto the handles, put your forearms on the arm rest, and keep your hips and torso against the back support. Without rocking or swaying your hips raise your feet up so that they're parallel to the floor. While your legs are parallel (this is the midpoint) squeeze your abs hard for one second. Then slowly lower your feet to the starting position. Repeat this until failure.

All three of these abdominal exercises work the abs in the exact same manner. You only need to do one exercise per day and only one set of that exercise.

Chapter Six:

Mindset.

I can't teach you how to lose a lot of weight fast without first teaching you about having the right mindset. Throughout my twenty-one years of being a Health & Fitness Professional I've learned how powerful having a positive mindset is for achieving your goals. You have to first believe that you can lose a lot of weight fast before you can actually do it. One of my favorite quotes to live by is:

*When I Believe It Then I'll See It! Remember that!

It is very possible to lose 30-50 pounds of bodyfat in only thirty days. I know because I've helped many people achieve these kinds of results. However, if you don't believe these kinds of results are possible then you'll never achieve these kinds of results. So, how can you increase your confidence and get results fast? Read on!

In order for you to lose weight fast the first thing you must have is the right mindset. A lot of people go to the gym and workout every single day, but very few have a lean and energetic physique. That's because only a few have the right mindset to build a sexy body that is admired on the beach. So, how do you train your mind properly? You train your mind by doing four things on a daily, ongoing, consistent basis.

1. You read books.

2. You listen to cd's.

3. You confess what you want.

4. You write out what you want.

You have to read books that inspire you, uplift you, and make you believe that you can do anything. Reading books on a daily basis will reprogram your mind. The more you read the stronger your mind will be. Here's a few of my all time favorite books that will help you reprogram your mind for success, rather than failure:

-The Holy Bible
-The Dream Giver
-The Power Of I Am
-The Attractor Factor
-Spirit Driven Success
-Think And Grow Rich
-Battlefield Of The Mind
-Transform Your Thinking
-The Magic Of Thinking Big
-The Power Of Positive Thinking

The second thing you need to do is listen to positive, uplifting audio cd's. You can buy cd's on the internet, or you can even listen to videos on YouTube. Every single night when my wife and I go to sleep we listen to something positive on YouTube and let it play all night long. The first thing in the morning when you wake up, and the last thing at night before you go to sleep are the most powerful times of the day for you to reprogram your mind for success. Some great speakers that my wife and I listen to on a regular basis are:

-Jim Rohn
-Les Brown
-Joel Osteen
-Bill Winston
-Rick Warren
-Jerry Savelle
-Creflo Dollar
-Dani Johnson
-Anthony Robbins
-Andrew Womack

The third thing you need to do is confess out loud exactly what you want in your life. Whatever it is that you want you need to speak positive words about it every single day. For example, if you want to lose fifty pounds you would say out loud all throughout the day something like this: I feel amazing now that I'm fifty pounds lighter. You will speak this affirmation out loud over and over throughout the day so that you can hear yourself saying it. By speaking it out loud and hearing yourself it will start to reprogram your mind.

The fourth thing you need to do is write down what you want to achieve. I have a notepad that I write affirmations in every single day and I encourage you to do the same. If you're going to do this you want to focus on one affirmation at a time until you achieve it. For example, if you want to lose fifty pounds you could write down throughout the day something like this: I feel amazing now that I'm fifty pounds lighter. You can write this down as many times as you want. The more you do it the faster it will start to reprogram your mind. I recommend that you write this down for about twenty-five times every single day until you achieve your goal of losing fifty pounds.

Doing these four things every single day will wash your brain clean from all the brain washing you've gone through in your life. Once you completely wash your brain clean from any bad programming that's been instilled in you, you'll then be able to manifest anything you want in life, including losing fifty pounds, sculpting a lean, sexy stomach, or having more energy. Train your mind and your body will follow.

Chapter Seven:

Junk Food.

Let me first go on record and say a stupid, common sense disclaimer, which I sure hope you already know: Yes, I eat junk food. Yes, I do splurge from time to time. Yes, it's possible to eat sugary, sweet desserts now and then and not get fat. I'm living proof of that!

However, I only eat these kinds of foods once or twice per week. That's it, nothing more! Surely, everyone knows you can't eat these kinds of foods every day and lose weight. Just in case you think you can eat like this every day and lose weight, let me be the first person to tell you- NO!

So, let me take a moment and share my secrets with you on how you can eat your favorite junk foods and not get fat. What I'm about to share with you I've been implementing myself for over twenty-one years now. That's why I can eat sugar filled, fattening foods and not get sad, worried, or depressed about gaining weight at all. I know that everything else that I do will keep these foods from making me fat. Follow these guidelines of mine and you'll be able to have your cake and eat it too.

-Only eat junk food for one or two of your meals per week. Eating more than this will make you fat and sick.

-On the days when you have a cheat meal you should eat less that day so your overall calorie count is lower for that day than usual. For example, I only eat three meals per day. However, on days when I have a cheat meal I'll only eat two meals. The reduction in my overall calories for that day will kind of balance out the bad calories that I ate. This will make sure the cheat meal that I ate will do the least amount of damage to my body fat levels.

Do an extra fifteen to thirty minutes of cardio the day after you have one of your cheat meals. This extra bit of cardio will burn off some of those extra calories you ate making sure they do the least amount of damage to your body fat levels.

Incorporate as many of my weight loss secrets as you possibly can. The more of my weight loss secrets that you incorporate on a consistent basis the less weight you will gain because you'll be reprogramming your body and metabolism to burn those bad calories off as soon as they digest.

I practice what I preach. Everything I've shared with you in this valuable book, I actually implement into my own life every single day. That's why I have single digit body fat levels every single day of the year. Once you start losing weight you'll increase your energy levels, increase your self-confidence, and increase your feelings of well-being. Since you've detoxed your body from healthy eating habits you won't crave junk foods anymore.

You will then only want to consume junk foods as a personal reward, or on a special occasion. When you eat junk foods sparingly you will not only feel better on the inside, but you'll look better on the outside as well.

Chapter Eight:

Weight Loss Challenge.

I want to finish by inviting you to a personal thirty-day Weight Loss Challenge! This is only between you and yourself. I've given you all the information you need to lose weight fast and get into the best shape of your life, but it's up to you to do it.

You have just learned all my best weight loss secrets. Now you've got to start incorporating them into your daily lifestyle like I have. You have to decide that right now is the time you're going to lose this weight and change your life once and for all. No more excuses! No more whining! No more complaining!

I've made a thirty-day calendar for you. I want you to write your current bodyweight inside of day one. Then I want you to weigh yourself again exactly one week later at the same time of day and on the same scale. This is for consistency. Weigh yourself just one time per week for the next thirty days for a total of four weigh-ins.

You need to be consistent for thirty days to see some good results. Like I said before, it is very possible to lose 30-50 pounds of bodyfat in only thirty days, but you have to be consistent in doing everything I shared with you in this book.

Put a red star on each day that you eat healthy, do your cardio, workout, and follow my powerful weight loss secrets. On the days that you don't follow through put a big black X. You want to have red stars not black X's. The more red stars you have the faster the weight is going to come off.

Everything you just learned in this book can change your health and life forever, if you'll follow it!

I can lead the horse to the water, but I can't make him drink. I just laid out everything you need to lose weight fast and get into the best shape of your life, but I can't make you do what I laid out for you. You have to do the work. You have to choose to change your life. You have to follow through on what you said you're going to do. When you get to your goal weight you'll feel so good about yourself. You deserve that! You took the first step by buying this book, now I encourage you to take the second step and get into the best shape of your life. Now, go do it!

Now that you've read this book, would you mind doing me a HUGE favor please? Would you be kind enough to write me a five-star customer review for this book on Amazon? By giving this book a five star review it will help me as an author and help more people be able to find the book on Amazon. Your words do have power. If you would be kind enough to write me a five star review for this book I would greatly appreciate it. I love hearing from people who have read my books. Please feel free to contact me any time. I wish you the very best of success in every area of your life!

Stacy Mitchell

www.ChangeYourLifeOvernight.com

If you enjoyed reading this book here's more books by the author:

1. True Story: Lies, Drugs, Abuse, Alcohol, Adultery, Illness, & Divorce!

2. Sell Your First Book!

3. Money Meditation Manifestation!

4. My Inspiring True Life Story!

5. How To Get Rich From Home On A Part Time Basis With Only $20!

6. The 6 Financial laws Of Success!

7. Why You're Fat & Sick And How To Fix It!

8. Faith Produces Miracles!

9. Entrepreneurship: Money, Wealth, & Prosperity!

All books can be purchased from:
www.amazon.com/author/fitchristophermitchell

1	2	3	4	5	6	7
8	9	10	11	12	13	14
15	16	17	18	19	20	21
22	23	24	25	26	27	28
29	30